HOMOEOPATHY IN
CANCER

by
PROF. DR. FAROKH JAMSHED MASTER
PROFESSOR OF MEDICINE, C.M.P.H. MEDICAL COLLEGE
BOMBAY UNIVERSITY.
HONORARY PHYSICIAN, BOMBAY HOSPITAL
HONORARY PHYSICIAN, K.E.M. HOSPITAL.
BOMBAY

B. JAIN PUBLISHERS (P) LTD.
USA — EUROPE — INDIA

HOMOEOPATHY IN CANCER

5th Impression: 2012

Published by Kuldeep Jain for

B. JAIN PUBLISHERS (P) LTD.
1921/10, Chuna Mandi, Paharganj, New Delhi 110 055 (INDIA)
Tel.: +91-11-4567 1000   Fax: +91-11-4567 1010
Email: info@bjain.com   Website: **www.bjain.com**

Printed in India by
J.J. Offset Printers

ISBN: 978-81-319-0721-4

PREFACE

I had an excellent opportunity to present a Scientific Paper viz. "THE HOMOEOPATHIC APPROACH TO CANCER" for my organizers, The Medical Institute for Homoeopathic Research and Application at Cyprus.

The Homoeopathic Profession has not seen for last 23 years any new therapeutic book on Cancer. The last was published by Dr. Fortier-Bernoville, M.D. A.H. Grimmer, M.D. in the year 1965. It was a difficult task for me to go through the literature and the past records of my patients of last 10 years.

In this booklet I have tried to make the difficult problem of the treatment of cancer patients much more easier. The Philosophical, including the maismatic background has been clearly explained with an easy understanding of some of the common as well as the rare remedies. I hope this little book will be found by my brother Homoeopaths as a useful collection in their library.

This work would have remained incomplete if I had not received encouragement and moral support from my learned teacher Dr. K.N. Kasad.

I also sincerely thank - Dr. Kamal Eruch Kodia for her assistance all throughout the publication of this book, Dr. Meherzin Noshir Dubash and Miss Roda Bandrawalla helped for preparation of Repertory and proof reading.

Last but not the least I sincerely thank Mr Kuldip and Premnath Jain of M/S B. Jain Publishers for printing this book at the most shortest notice.

Vatcha Gandhi Memorial   —DR. FAROKH J. MASTER
Building No. 1
Hughes Road
Bombay - 400 007

THE HOMOEOPATHIC APPROACH TO CANCER

INTRODUCTION

The last few years have witnessed remarkable progress in understanding the biologic and biochemical bases for cancer.

This is not to imply that the problem of neoplastic disease is solved, because despite in surgery, chemotherapy, and radiation therapy, cancer accounts for fourth of all deaths in the United States each year.

This paper provides on overview of the definition, etiology, Miasmatic aspects, Homoeopathic treatment followed by a description of the anthroposophical drugs.

Definition

The disease called cancer is best defined by four characteristics which describe how cancer cells act differently from their normal counter parts.

a) **Clonality** : In most cases, cancer originates from a single stem cell which proliferates to form a clone of malignant cells.

b) **Autonomy** : Growth is not properly regulated by the normal biochemical and physical influences in the environment.

c) **Anaplastic** : There is lack of normal coordinated cell differentiation.

d) **Metastasis** : Cancer cells developed the capacity for discontinuous growth and dissemination to other parts of the body.

Philosophy of Tumor Cell Biology

Since all cells in an organism originate from single fertilized egg (Zygote), all carry the identical genetic information. The proliferation and differentiation of this cell into an embryo, and eventually into a mature organism, involve selective and co-ordinated expression of the genomic repertoire control of gene expression is accomplished through incompletely understood molecular interactions which can be modulated, in part, by chemical influences in the environment.

The genomic repertoire includes information which permits cells to expand clonally, to function with varying degrees of autonomy, to differentiate and dedifferentiate, and to move from one part of the organism to another in a co-ordinated way.

In the adults the process of wound healing activates expression of these cellular characteristics in a more "embryo-like" fashion, but under well co-ordinated control. In the case of malignancy, the normal control process is subverted or by passed due to the anomalous activities of a select group of genes (onco genes) which have central importance to the regulation of cellular activities.

THE MIASMATIC ASPECTS OF CANCER

Any disease has an evolution of miasmatic phase from Psora to Syphilis, the same holds true for cancer. Hahnemann in his chronic diseases classifies cancer under Psora (here actually he means the earliest precancerous states). Robert in his Principles & Art of Cure mentions cancer as multi-miasmatic. I would like to classify as follows : (1) All exophytic growths e.g. Warts, Dermoid cyst, Bony tumors, etc. are sycosyphilitic in nature. (2) All ulcerative and fungative growths are syphilitic in nature. (3) Whenever cancer is accompanied by haemorrahage and secondary infection it is due to presence of strong tubercular miasm.

What constitutes the fundamental cause?

In series of patients (approx. 100) treated by Dr. Kasad from India, demonstrated to us that family or past history of cancer, Pulmonary tuberculosis and Diabetes are the frequent findings in the cases of cancer which clearly confirms that cancer in a patient develops, on the platform of strong syco-syphilitic affections. when there is a strong family history of cancer or T.B. then there are chances either in first or second generations where one finds cases of cancer in the infancy like Acute Lymphatic Leukemia, etc.

To use the language of Dr. A.H. Grimmer I quote "My experience has been that there is not a case of Cancer without a tubercular background. It growths on a tubercular soil. It is the miasm where in the blending of all the other miasms results."

In my personal series of approximately 32 patients I have observed that in the family and past history of cancer patients there is a marked predominance of Diabetes, Coronary artery disease, Hypertension, Degenerative Joint Diseases, Cancer and Cerebro Vascular Accident.

What constitutes the precipitating cause ?

The following precipitating cause have been frequently observed in cases of cancer :

(1) The emotional trauma, grief reactions; precautionary losses; bereavements, mental stress and strain.

(2) **Radiation :** Information on the capacity of radiation in relatively large doses to induce cancer in humans comes from studies on survivors of atomic bomb blast, on individuals accidentally exposed to irradiation, on patients exposed to radiations for diagnostic purposes.

(3) **Tobacco :** Numerous epidemiologic studies have demonstrated that principle carcinogenic agent in our environment is inhaled tobacco smoke. The incidence of lung cancer is more than tenfold higher in, male smokers than in non-smokers.

(4) **Occupational exposure :** The first report of cancer related to occupational hazards was Percival Pott's observation of an unusually high frequency of scrotal cancer among London chimney sweeps. The following table provides a partial listing of industrial agents which are known to cause cancer.

Etiology	Site of Malignancy
Arsenic	Lung, Skin, Liver
Asbestos	Mesolthelium, Lung
Benzene	Leukemia
Benzidine	Bladder
Chromium Compounds	Lung
Radiation	Numerous location

4

Etiology	Site of Malignancy
Mustard gas	Lung
Ploycyclic Hydro carbons	Lung, Skin
Vinyl Chloride	Angio-sacoma of the liver

Selection of Remedy

Selecting a remedy in a case of cancer should be on constitutional basis i.e. to consider the mental, physical generals, physical particulars, aggravation and amelioration factors including life situation. Unfortunately one cannot follow the above procedure because of following reasons ;

1. Patient comes to us fairly late in his sickness i.e. with distant metastasis.

2. By the time he sees us he has already taken enough suppressive measure like surgery, chemotherapy and radiation.

Repetitive Suppressive measure in the past pushes the constitutional symptoms in the background as a result on the surface one gets a maze of non-characteristic, pathological, non peculiar symptoms. Hence the principle in prescribing in such cases should be purely palliative.

1. **Patients who present in a pre-cancerous condition or in the most earliest stage**

The above group of patients stand a good chance of cure. A careful prescribing in such cases helps us to remove the disease from the root. Selection of a deep–acting constitutional remedy based on the patient's mental state, physical generals, modalities and particulars. One should start with a medium of potency (200 or 500) with frequent repetition till the time one gets the desired result. Intercurrent remedies like nosodes should always be included so as to clear the path for the remedies to act.

Since it is the beginning of the illness the susceptability of the patient is quite high and the case is full of peculiar, queer, uncommon symptoms. Hence, the chances of cure is maximum. Sometimes it may happen whilst giving a constitutional remedy in a high potency (10M, 50M, CM) with frequent repetition one may have a temporary phase of frightful aggravation. This is considered to be a positive response and it indicates that one should stop further administration of the remedy and to wait and watch.

2. **Patients who present with advanced cancer with distant metastasis**

In the above cases one finds the picture is purely pathological. There is absence of peculiar, queer and uncommon symptoms. The susceptibility is extremely low. Hence one should be extremely careful about giving a potency too high with frequent repetition. I prefer a low potency, say the 6X 12X or 30X. One gets better results and one can easily avoid those terrible aggravation of the higher potencies. However, I may add over here that in many cases of advanced malignancy, I had occasion to observe constitutional as well as peculiar, queer and uncommon symptom, as for example, "Burning pain in throat with desire for ice cold drinks"—an indication for phosphorus in an advanced case of cancer of Pyriform fossa. Phosporus 30 was selected for the patient and only one dose was administered. The patient agony and discomfort were greatly ameliorated. On the fourth day the patient expired. This clearly demonstrated Homoeopathic palliation.

It is extremely important for a young physician to know how to judge the susceptibility of the individual. In an advance case of the cancer the following guidelines are extremely useful :

1. Feeling of well-being.
2. Vital signs like pulses, B.P., temperature and Respiratory rate.
3. Good appetite.
4. Bladder/bowel function including intake and output being normal.
5. Absence of electrolyte imbalance.
6. Absence of anaemia.

All the above points indicate a good susceptibility. In such a case even though there is presence of pathological symptoms one can select a deep–acting constitutional remedy in a higher potency with fre-

frequent repetition as such patients do not develop a severe aggravation. This requires an efficient moniteering of the patient and his symptoms including a rigid regular medical examination with investigations.

Treatment of Pre-cancerous state

One should be well aware that following pre-cancerous state does occur such as :

1. Ulcerative colitis
2. Cervical erosion (paparicolaou III & IV)
3. Kraurosis valvae
4. Leukoplakia
5. Proliferative mastopathy St. III

6. Crohn's disease.
7. Papillomatosis of the bladder
8. Intestinal plyposis
9. Chronic gastric ulcer
10. Seborrhoeic keratosis.

In such a situation one should enquire for any cancer cases in the family. Also past family history of Syphilis, gonorrhoea or T.B. should be inquired. Further history of repeated vaccination should be inquired. Do there exists certain signs of pre-cancerous state such as, yellow spots on the skin, naevi (signs of Thuja), or again, a disturbed mental state through the morbid fear of cancer? (Arsenic, Calacarea, Psorinum). Symptoms like weakness, anaemia, pallor, loss of weight, change in bowel habit in an elderly person, should be strongly considered as a symptom of overt cancer.

Treatment should consist in the prescription of the constitutional remedy. Results will be excellent in most of the cases but one cannot depend on this for they are isolated accomplishment.

General Treatment of Cancer

This is composed of ;

1. Constitutional remedies.
2. Cancer remedies.
3. Drainage remedies.
4. Specific nosodes.
5. Anthroposophical remedies.

1. Constitutional Remedies

The following polycrest are quite often indicated in cancerous and pre-cancerous patients. My object over here only a practical one, viz. to present the general indication of some common constitutional remedies.

1. THUJA OCCIDENTALIS

Thuja occidentalis, the so called Arbor Vitae, is an evergreen conifer. This drug has a strong affinity with epithelial tissue, its irritantaction leading to oversecretion by glandular cells and hyperplasia of epithelium with formation of warty of condylomatous growths.

A heavy trunk, short neck, thin limbs, waxy greasy skin and irregular teeth are listed as characteristics of the Thuja subject, and in general a sickly look.

Excessive hairiness will be present in a women with a growth of a mostache and dark hair on the limbs. Obesity may be excessive. Movements tend to be unnaturally active and hurried. Hands are cold clammy to touch. Speech is either hesitant or hurried.

Discharge are copious, foul smelling, often greenish and thin, peculiar odour may suggest fish brine, garlic or honey.

Psychologically, there is a tendency to feel dazed, confused especially on walking from sleep. Fixed ideas may obtrude—"His soul is separated from his body"—"strange people is standing beside the bed" "Is pregnant"—"something alive is moving around in the belly"—"legs are made of wood". One peculiar odd sensation is of brittleness and liability to shatter in two little fragments. There is great sensitive to people, "atmosphere", and music. The patient is apathetic, desiring to be left alone; is ill-humoured, peevish, lachrymous—music may provoke tears.

The Thuja subject is unduly chilly and may shiver all over on exposure of the body even to warm air.

There is carving for salt and preference for cold food; there is a dislike of raw food and potatoes, and intolerance of onions. Thirst is not marked, it is said that fluids when swallowed drop into the stomach with a gurgling sound. The sleep is disturbed by anxious, amorous, sometimes frightful dreams, often of falling from a height. Profuse sweats occur on uncovered parts only. Thuja is a deeply acting remedy and should not be repeated too frequently. It may be of service at times in actue conditions. It should be considered when there is a history of gonorrhoea or herpes. Other etiological factors pointing to the possible views of Thuja in a case of cancer are :

1. Vaccination with severe reaction
2. Repeated unsuccessful vaccination
3. Serum injections
4. Excessive tea drinking.

Its complementary remedies are:

Lachesis, Medorrhinum, Silica and *Sycoti. Co.*

2. LACHESIS

This is prepared from the venom of lachesis muta.

The main affinity of the position is with the blood causing disintigration of the red cells. Lowered coagulity after initial tendency to thrombosis, and impaired resistence to infection with associated liability to gangrene and neurosis. Hence, it is used in cases of homoeopatic malignancies like leukaemia, etc.

The Lachesis patient is usually dark, spare, with a pale complexion. The face may acquire a purplish and bloated or red, congested, swollen appearance. The expression is anxious, suspicious even furtive, and the eyes wide as if with fear. The speech is torrential, logorrhoeic, spate, or may be slow and hesitant. Other physical signs that may be present are—shinny tongue with a "varnished" look, spontaneous bruising, purplish discolouration and foul smelling discharges.

The emotional feature of Lachesis subject are characteristic liable to be self conscious, selfish, conceited, jealous even suspicious without case. There is often an urge to confess crimes never committed. Unbearable anguish may assail especially on waking from sleep. Great sensitivity to all stimuli, but specially to touch and noise.

This is also a constitutional remedy of the first order for the precancerous and starting cancer cases. This is especially so in females approaching the fifth decade, following a period of glandular and circulatory disturbances affecting the thyroid, ovaries, and liver. These disturbances are often accomplished by vertigo, flushes of heat, palpitations, general hyperaesthesia (cannot tolerate anything tied about the neck, chest or waist) and often, arterial hypertension. If these exists a bloody discharge, the latter ameliorates the patient (especially the periods). If, on the other hand, there is cessation of the discharge the condition is aggravated (menopause).

There is susceptibility to either extremes of temperature but especially to heat.

3. IODIUM

The Iodium subject is dark hair, dark eyes, dark skin. The Idoium subject is restless, apprehensive, pre-occupied, anxious even anguished and expects the worst, is excessively impatient. There is tendency to impulsiveness, impulse to do something violent.

Again, the Iodium person may be zealous, literary, over-careful.

The Iodium subject is essentially a warm blooded type, wants a cool place to move, think and work in.

The Iodium patient is debilitated, weak, wastes very rapidly inspite of his good appetite. He has tendency to produce new connective tissues and hard gladular growths (breasts, uterus, lymphatic glands, thyroid, etc.) One must not neglect to prescribe it for it often has a favourable action on the weight and even on the tumoral element which it can cause to regress or whose induration and invasive tendency it will diminish.

Iodium is complementary to *Thuja* which is also its antidote.

4. SILICA

The Silica patient appears swallow, sickly, shivery, sweaty, suffering and small for its age. The head seems to large for the body and the belly too prominent. Psychologically, the Silica person is self-willed, touchy, full of apprehension. He lacks confidence in himself.

There is lack of "go" of "drive", of "gift", of "initiative" scrupulously consciencious, however, but lacking in application as thoughts tend to wander.

The person is timid, full of fears, especially a dread of failure from a feeling of incapacity.

"*Silica* is the remedy of depth for the overworked individual whose nervous resistance is used up. In this mistakes in speaking, talking and writing."

Chilliness predominates the picture. The appetite is poor. There is a desire for cold food and cold milk. Excessive thirst is the rule. There is presence of drenching sweat on the head and feet.

The remedy has a scrofulous diathesis as a result, it has an action on the various lymph modes. Hence, is used in various lymphomas and other malignances where lymph node is involved.

I have personally used this drug with great success in various cases of the non-healing of wounds post operatively for malignant patients where the offensive, thin, watery pus oozes out from the wound. The patient feels locally better by application warm packs.

The remedy also possesses an ability to stimulate an absorption of fibrosed and scar tissues. It should, therefore, be avoided in old cases of pulmonary T.B.

A remarkable feature of *Silica* is its ability to promote expulsion, exteriorization, foreign bodies from the tissues.

Silica is quite incompatible with Mercurius, and the two remedies should never be given near one another in point of time.

5. LYCOPODIUM

Lycopodium subject who becomes cancerous will localize his tumor preferentially on the liver, stomach, kidney or intestine. Lycopodium patients tend to have a sallow complexion often with flushed cheeks and a rather red nose. They appear lean, even emaciated, about the face, neck and chest, but are quite well covered in the lower part of the body. The brow tends to be wrinkled, with a marked vertical frown about root of the nose.

The head hair is plentiful, but body hair is scanty and the belly smooth. Early graying of the hair may occur. A peculiar physical sign that may be present is marked coldness of one foot while the opposite member is warm or hot.

Psychologically the patient is conscientious and orderly, he cannot bear to be corrected or opposed. He is intellectually active, must be occupied, finds relief in action, movement and active excercise. He is extremely self-conscious, shuns crowds, but is also averse to complete solitude and likes to have someone around. He is apprehensive before an ordeal, from defidence and lack of self confidence, but rises to the occasion when it arrives. He is fearful of the dark, of failure, from appearing in public.

A noticeable attribute is lack of aptitude for finance and commerce, not good either argument or arthmetic.

A definitely chilly individual. Hates the cold and feels paralysed thereby in both mind and muscle. At the same time he also tends to flag is great heat.

Appetitie is apt to be capricious. Starts a meal quite hungry but feels satisfied over a few mouthful. In the matter of food preferences and dislikes, there is a definite fondness for sugar and sweet things and marked preference for hot meals and hot fluids, also for scvaries. There is a tendency to eat too fast. There is intolerance of cabbage, peas, beans, milk, pastry, onions, oysters which tend to upset the digestion.

May perspire on slightest exertion—a cold clammy sweat with odour of onions.

The symptoms usually tend to be right sided and then extended to left.

Flatulent dyspepsia becomes an important concomitant with most of the Lycopodium complaints.

6. THE CALCAREAS

Of the three great calcium salts, calcarea fluor is the only one which exhibits a neoplastic element. It confers on glands or connective tissue—a stony induration (Conium, Carbo animalis). It acts as well in breast, bone and uterine cancer.

Calcarea phos has hardly any action on cancer or pre-cancerous states.

Calcarea carb is rather indicated among the pre-cancerous hypothyroids, hypersensitive to cold and chilly with flaccid muscles and integuments, malnourished, invaded by adipose tissue. The subject wastes rapidly after an initial phase of false plethora and fatty invasion. It can act selectively on the glandular hypertrophy.

Calcarea iodide will be indicated in suspicious and indolent ulceration with engorgement of lymph glands.

Calcarea oxalata should act on the pains in ulcerating cancers.

7. THE KALIS

Pre-cancerous cases often require *Kali carb* with symptoms like weakness, chills, lumbar pains, sweats, wasting.

Kali bichromicum is indicated when gastric or pyloric ulcer develops into malignant degeneration or there is presence of sluggish, indolent ulcerations with perpendicular borders with characteristic yellow, stringy, profuse discharge.

Kali iodide—among all the Kalis this syphilitic Kali has a selective action on the infilterated connective tissue, especially when associated with hypertrophied glands.

Kali ars is useful in inveterate skin disease with fissures and malignant tendency.

Kali cynatum is used in lingual cancer.

8. THE CARBOS

Carbo vegetabilis, for deficient vitality, for deficient oxygenation and nutrition, presenting a gastro-intestinal atony already old and stubborn, may be indicated in cancer (especially digestive) or the pre-cancerous state.

Carbo animalis is one of the best remedies for the established tumor; hard tumour; indurated and swollen lymphatic glands, subcutaneious venous distention, bluish discolouration of infiltrated tissues, burning pains, gastric flatulence. It has a special selective action on the breast and stomach cancer and merits special mention not only for its beneficial effects on the general state (gain of weight or temporary arrest of wasting) but also for its action on the tumor itself which regresses, becomes less hard with amelioration of pains.

9. CAUSTICUM

The Causticum subject is liable to have dark hair, dark eyes, pale skin. There is makred restlessness with inability to lie still. In speech there is a tendency to stammer or make spunerism.

Psychologically Causticum patient is described as unhappy, weepy, hopeless, timid, nervous and anxious. Is easily upset emotionally and may become hysterical.

Is full of foreboding and apprehension with great fear of darkness. There is a tendency to become peevish, irritable, censorious or suspicious. A feature may be intense and sympathy with the sufferings of other people. It is worthy to note that causticum malignancy may derive from sudden emotional stress or from long lasting grief or worry.

The Causticum person is chilly, but also averse to either extreme of temperature.

Appetite is capricious; sits down to a meal quite hungry, but the thought, smell, even sight of food, takes away all desire. There is an aversion to sweet things, and a desire rather for pungent delicacies.

Despite a burning thirst for cold drinks, especially beer, the subject may shrink from the act of drinking.

10. NITRIC ACID

This remedy has a profound action on the various cells of the human tissue producing multiple sycosyphilitic affections. The acid possesses a destructive ulcerating affinity on mucocutaneous junction (oral cavity, anus) resulting in development of cracks and fissures ultimately leading to malignant changes.

The face appears pale, pinched, with sallow complexion and dark rings around the orbits. The subject is likely to be emanciated with obvious weakness manifested by a constant desire to sit or lie down. The limbs show tremors or twitching of muscles.

Discharges offensive, thin, excoriating and possibly of a dirty yellowishgreen colour.

Psychologically the patient is depressed and anxious, especially in the evening, worries about disease with fear of death.

The patient is easily startled and is intolerant of sympathy at the same time is extremely hypersensitive to touch, pain, noise or jar. The patient is obstinate, taciturn and may exhibit vindictiveness. The memory is poor and thoughts vanish when attempting to concentrate.

Physiologically the patient is chilly and shivery even near the fire; the patient has cold hands and feet. There is craving for both fats and salt. Occasionally there could be perversion of appetite with a desire for chalk, lime, earth. Bread always disagrees with the patient.

The patient tends to be drowsy during the day. There is profuse sweat on hands and feet and sweets are very exhausting and malodourous. The most prominent feature is extreme weakness and cachexia.

Peculiar sharp splinter-like pain which comes and goes suddenly. Those peculiar pains are touch off by contact, by movement, when swallowing, when passing a stool or from contact or dressings with the surface of an ulcer.

Haemorrhages are apt to occur from any mucous surface and are usually of bright red blood.

11. ARSENICUM ALBUM

Very important and often indicated, arsenicum, by its prostration alternating or coexisting with a certain agitation, by its burning pains, ameliorated by heat, its characteristic horary, clearly individualizes many confirmed cancer cases to whom it will often bring a temporary amelioration, transitory or slightly prolonged, as in very weak cancerous subjects.

Such are the principal constitutional remedies we ought to review. The dilutions in which they ought to be employed are variable enough. In a general way, the high potencies will be reserved for the precancerous state; the low and middle potencies for the confirmed cancers.

Let us hasten to add that the results obtained with these remedies alone are very uncertain, the cases of real cure are very rare; simple amelioration very variable in confirmed neoplasms. On the other hand, in multiple precancer cases success is frequent.

II. CANCER REMEDIES

There are numerous remedies for cancer in Homoeopathy. Here I have selected few out of the group as I have confirmed its clinical use in my practice or have read about it in the scientific journal. For the sake of convenience, I have classified these remedies into various groups :

(I) The Most Habitual Remedies

These are the ones which have revealed themselves as having the most constant action on the tumoral element as well as the general state.

1. SEDUM ACRE AND SEDUM REPENS

In material doses, other tincture, 1X and 3X. it has an undeniable action on cancer in general, gives weight to the patients, and occasionally modifies the tumor, or at least retards its progress. Their principle sign is their tendency to mucosal and cutaneous fissures which are so frequent in cancer or the precancerous state. The pathogenesis of these two remedies is incomplete. Because of that we must be satisfied to use them in an empericle fashion. Sedum Teleplium, another plant of the same family, should act especially on the uterus or cancerous rectum with haemorrhages.

2. SEROFULARIA NODOSA

This remedy acts especially on cancers of breast, skin, uterus, rectum, in low potencies or material doses, especially if there is marked glandular invasion.

3. SEMPERVIVUM TECTORUM

Lingual, breast, rectal and other cancers. Its tendency to apthae, to malignant ulcers, specially indicates it in the ulcerated cancer. It must also be used in mother tincture or low potencies.

4. CONDURAGO

I have personally observed the value of *Condurango* in oesophageal, stomach or intestinal cancers. One if its valuable external signs consists in fissures of the labial commissues. It also acts on cancer situated at the junction of mucosa and skin, lips, anus, lids.

5. CISTUS CANADENSIS

This remedy acts especially in cancer of the breast, pharynx or neck and gives rise to very marked cervical adenopathy.

6. HYDRASTIS

As good for the breast as for the stomach, Hydrastis is of great value in cancer, ulcerated or not, with progressive debility, wasting emaciation, hypochlorhydria is frequent before and during the phase of gastric ulcer.

7. KRESOTUM

Bleeding ulcerations, vegetations develop reapidly and emit a burning discharge, excoriating, fetid; such are the principal signs of *Kreosote* which acts especially well in cancer of cervix.

8. ORNITHOGALUM

This remedy has a remarkable action on the pylorodeuodenal sphere. Its main use is in cases which are associated with vomitting of coffee ground colour. There is presence of pain in the stomach which increases when passes through the pyloric outlet.

9. PHYTOLACCA

Chiefly used for hard and scirrhous tumor of the breast. The mammae are hard and extremely sensitive with enlarged axillary glands. Presence of irritable before and during menses with dominant syphilitic miasm confirms the picture.

(II) Remedies for Pain

1. ARSENIC ALBUM

Pains are maddening, burns like fire. Pains are better by local appliacation of heat, pain causes shortness of breath or chilliness. Sudden great weakness with restlessness are important concomitant.

2. APIS MELLIFICA

Burning, stinging pricks as with red hot needles associated with numbness, shinny red discolouration. Especially useful for relieving pains that arise from Carcinoma of the tongue, breast, larynx and ovary.

3. ARNICA

Bruise pain which arises from the cancerous part associated with echymotic blue black spots following traumatism. Chiefly used in cases of benign and malignant tumor of the breast.

4. BRYONIA:

The pains are bursting, stitching or heavy sore; going backwards. Effects are very painful. On coughing holds, sides, chest, head, associated with streaks of red-lymphangitis. Chiefly used for breast cancer which ought to be supported or bound.

5. CALCAREA ACETICUM

Chiefly useful for excruciating, constricting pains of cancer.

6. EUPHORBIUM

There is extreme sensation of burning with lancinating pain, especially in bones at night. Chiefly useful for relieving the pain of osteogenic sarcoma and multiple myeloma.

7. MAGNESIUM PHOS

Neuralgic pains which are sharp shooting like lightning, suddenly changing places; radiating, boring, constricting, extorting cries; causing restlessness and prostration, etc.

The pains relieved by warmth, pressure and rubbing.

8. RUTA

The pains are bruised, sore, aching with restlessness, especially arising from osseous or periosteal tissue. There is presence of intense weakness. The selective sphere of actions are bone, periostem, cartilage, rectum.

(III) Organ and Rare Remedies

It has clinical confirmation of its use in cancerous ulcers and modulated tumors of the tongue.

1. GALIUM APARINE

It has a specific action on the urinary organs producing diuresis.

2. FULIGO LIGNI

It is useful in epithelioma of the skin and for cancer expecially of scrotum and uterus. It is also used for obstinate non-healing malignant ulcers of the skin.

3. KREOSOTUM

Follows extremely well after *FULIGO LIGNI*.

4. HOANG NAN

It is capable of ameliorating the fetidy and haemorrhages of cancer by causing an improvement in the general condition. It is especially indicated in cancer of the glandular structures.

5. CINANMONUM

It is especially indicated in cancer when pain and fetor are present. It is useful in haemorrhages which are bright red in colour.

6. ANATHERUM

It is useful in induration of breasts, tongue and cervix characterized by ulceration, inflammation and enlargement of lymphglands.

7. CHOLINE

Choline is a constituent of Taraxacum root. It has given a encouraging result in the treatment of cancer especially through its action on the liver.

8. CHOLESTERINUM

It is used for cancer of liver where presence of gaundice or gall stones are important pathological findings.

9. EOSIN

It is useful for burning pain of cancer as reported by Dr. B. C. Woodbury.

10. RADIUM BROMIDE

It is used for cutaneous epitheliomata and as an antidote for bad effects of X-Ray irradiation in a patient who has been treated too intensely. It is also used in cases of ulcers due to radium burns which take a long time to heal.

11. X-RAY

It is usually indicated in cases of cancer following skin lesions produced by repeated exposure to X-Ray. X-Ray is also used in cases of Leukaemia. It antidotes the unfortunate effects of radium in patients who have been treated by it.

(IV) Drainage Remedies

Dr. Nebel, had postulated that eliminating or neutilizing toxins that arises from the cancer tissue should be drained from the body similarly essential mineral salts should be added to the body to prevent malnutrition.

In other words drainage ought to be directed if possible, via the local selective action of certain well individualized remedies.

Given below is the chart of local selective action of Homoeopathic remedies in cancer. I have prepared the table and it is always open for any further additions or modifications.

1. LIPS : Condurango, Con, Carb-an, Kali-ar.
2. PALATE : Canth, Hydr, Aur.
3. TONGUE : Kali cyantum, Sempervirum tectorum, Galium, Aparine.
4. PHARYNX : Cistus candensis.
5. OESOPHAGUS : Condurango.
6. STOMACH : Carbo animalis, Condurango, Hydrastis, Lycopodium, Kali bichromicum.

7. PYLORUS AND DUODENUM : Ornithogalum.

8. INTESTINES : Condurango, Carbo—ani, Ars alb, Sedum repens, Petroleum.

9. CAECUM : Ornithogalum.

10. SIGMOID COLON AND RECTUM : Ruta, Scrofularia Nodosa, Sempervirum tectorum, Alum, Nit-ac, Ruta, Sep, Hydr, Kalicyan.

11. ANUS : Condurago.

12. LIVER : Cholesterinum, Lycopodium, Phosphorus, Choline.

13. PANCREAS : Phosphorus.

14. UTERUS : Phos, Sep, Sil, Aurum mur, Thuja, Natronatum, Kreosotum, Ars, Ars-i, Con, Elaps, Graph, Hydr, Lach, Lyco, Murex.

15. BREASTS : Asterias, Rubens, Conium, Carbo—ani, Hydrastis, Sempervirum Tectorum, Carcinosin, Bufo, Graph, Merc, Sil.,

16. TESTICLES : Aurum met, Spong.

17. SCROTUM : Fuligo ligni, Carb-an, Ph-ac.

18. SKIN : Sacrofularia nodosa, Condurango, Galium aparine, Ars. alb, Thuja, Cinnabaris, Petroleum, Kali-ars, Rad—brom,

19. EYE : Condurango. Aurum, Calc, Lyco, Phos, Sep, Sil, Thuja.

20. PERIOSTEUM : Ruta, Sympahytum, Phosphorus.

21. LYMPHATIC GANDS IN GENERAL : Carbo animalis.

22. GLANDS IN GENERAL : Scrofularia nodosa, Iodium, Calc. fluorica, Calc (parotid), Aurm, Carbm, Carb—an, Con, Buni-O, Sieg, Stynch-g, Sul-i, Syph.

23. FACE : Thuja, Cinnabaris.

24. NECK : Cistus canadensis, Merc (parotids).

26. VAGINA : Kreos.

26. BLADDER : Taraxac.

27. AXILLA : Asteria rubens.

(V) Specific Nosodes:

It is always advisable to prescribe nosodes on symptom similarity rather than prescribing emperically. In a given case the predisposing miasm along with the dominant miasm should be considered and respective nosodes like *Tuberculinum*, *Medorhinum* or *Syphilinum* should be prescribed.

1. CARCINOSIN

I had opportunity to use *Carcinosin* very frequently in my practice in cases where there is a strong family history of cancer.

Dr. D.M. Foubistr in the year 1954-58 had given us a descriptive picture of the drug carcinosin. I quote "The subject have a bluish tinge to the sclera, a brownish cafe-au-lait complexion, many pigmented moles".

Psychologically, the subject may be fatidious, is sensitive to music and has prolonged fear with worry and anticipation.

These patients are always better by taking a short nap. There is strong craving for salt, milk, egg and fat.

Secretions in general may be acrid and thick.

Preparation of Carcinosin

The original preparation previously known as Carcinosium and used by Kent, Burnett, and Clarke is thought to have been prepared from a breast epithelioma. It is this preparation which will be dispensed if the prescriber simply writes Carcinosin. However a number of new varieties of carcinosin has been prepared from specimens obtained from the operating theatre of the Royal London Homoeopathic Hospital. They are as follows :

Preparation	Origin
Carcinosin Adeno.Stom	Epithelioma of Stomach
Carcinosin Adeno Vesica	Epithelioma of Bladder
Carcinosin Intest. Co	Epithelioma of Intestine and Bladder
Carcinosin Scin. Mam	Scirrus of Breast
Carcinosin Squam. Pulm.	Epithelioma of Lung

Their drug pictures have not been differentiated, and it would seem that a strong family history of one of the above may be a pointer to its use.

2. BOWEL NOSODES

In U.K. Dr. Bach and Dr. Dishington have used their nosodes taken from cultures of intestinal organisms which are nonlactose fermenters; Gaertner, Morgan, Dysentericus, Proteus, are proposed. Here are their indications :

In carcinoma : Morgan and Dysentericus.

In sarcoma : Morgan and Gaertner.

(VI) Anthroposophical Remedies

Starting from philosophical and metaphysical ideas, Rudolf Steiner noted that the mistletoe (Viscum album) ought to be a real specific remedy in cancer.

Composition : A fermented aqueous extract of viscum ablum from different host trees processed by a special method.

Uses : Malignant diseases and Precancerous states.

Mode of action

A number of preclinical studies have indicated that *Viscum* album stimulates an immune response at cellular level. Other researches suggest selective damage to tumour cells.

The specific action of *Viscum album* is by activating defence mechanism and consequently tumor inhibition, is evident from the following effects commonly seen in cancer patients given *Viscum album* for cancer:

(a) Improvement in general condition.

(b) Improved appetite and weight gain.

(c) Better sleep.

(d) Relief of tiredness and depression.

(e) Improved urinary and bowel function.

(f) Slowing down and cessation of tumour growth.

(g) Occasional regression of tumours.

(h) Reduced incidence of metastasis.

CONCLUSION

Without hoping for too much with absolute tenacity let us treat established cancer cases. If we can almost never cure it, let us be able to hope in obtaining a certain equilibrium, which is more or less stable between the patient and his disease. Fused with deligence patience and tenacity, such is what we hope to achieve without patients suffering from cancer, and for that matter any other disease.

BIBLIOGRAPHY

1. **PRINCIPLES OF NEOPLASIA**

    - JOHN MENDELSOHN
      HARRISON'S PRINCIPLES OF INTERNAL MEDICINE 1
      ELEVENTH EDITION

    - **Edited by -**   BRAUNWALD
                          ISSELBACHER
                          PETERSDORF
                          WILSON
                          MARTIN
                          FAUCI

    - **Published by -** Mc Graw Hill
                           Health Profession Series

2. **PRINCIPLES OF CANCER THERAPY**

    - VINCENT T. DEVITA, JR.
      HARRISON'S PRINCIPLES OF INTERNAL MEDICINE 1
      ELEVENTH EDITION

    - **Edited by -**   BRAUNWALD
                            ISSEL BACHER
                          PETERSDORF
                          WILSON
                          MARTIN
                          FAUCI

    - **Published by-** Mc Graw Hill
                           Health Profession Series

3. **INTENSIVE CARE OF THE CANCER PATIENT**

        GRAZIANO C. CARLON, M.D.
        ALAN D. TURNBULL, M.D.
        WILLIAM S. HOWLAND, M.D.

4. **TERMINAL CARE**

C.M. SAUNDERS
OXFORD TEXT BOOK OF MEDICINE
Vol II : Section 13-28, Appendix and Index

Edited by - D.J. WEATHERALL
J.G.G. LEDINGHAM
D.A. WARRELL

SECOND EDITION
Published by - ELBS

5. **REPERTORY OF THE HOMOEOPATHICH MATERIA MEDICA**

by - J.T. KENT, A.M., M.D.

Published by - B. JAIN PUBLISHERS (P) Ltd.

6. **STUDIES OF HOMOEOPATHIC REMEDIES**

- DOUGLAS M. GIBSON
M.B., B.S. (Lond.), FRCS (Edin.),
FF Hom.

Edited by - DR. MARIANNE HARLING
BA, BM, BCh, FF Hom.
DR. BRIAN KAPLAN
MB, Bch, MF Hom.

7. **HOMOEOPATHIC TREATMENT OF CANCER**

by - FORTIER - BERNOVILLE, M.D.
&
A.H. GRIMMER, M.D.

Published by - B. JAIN PUBLISHERS (P) Ltd.

8. **POCKET MANUAL OF HOMOEOPATHIC MATERIA MEDICA**

by - WILLIAM BOERICKE, M.D.
NINTH EDITION

Published by - B. JAIN PUBLISHERS (P) Ltd,

9. **SYNTHETIC REPERTORY**

Published by - B. JAIN PUBLISHERS (P) Ltd.

Psychic and General Symptoms of the Homoeopathic Materia Medica

Vol I -   Mental Symptoms
Vol II -   General Symptoms
Vol III - Sleeping and Sexual Symptoms

10. **A DICTIONARY OF PRACTICAL MATERIA MEDICA**

CLARKE

Published by - B. JAIN PUBLISHERS (P) Ltd,

Vol I
Vol II
Vol III

11. **ISCADOR THERAPY**

SYMPOSIUM VOLUME
J.C.R.
DR. K.N. KASAD

12. **THE PRINCIPLES AND ART OF CURE BY HOMOEOPATHY**

- HERBERT A. ROBERTS, M.D.

- Published by-B. Jain Publishers (P) Ltd.